Rivelino Portes Ribeiro

Compulsory Notification of Violence in Primary Health Care

Rivelino Portes Ribeiro

Compulsory Notification of Violence in Primary Health Care

What health professionals say

ScienciaScripts

Cover image: www.ingimage.com

This book is a translation from the original published under ISBN 978-613-9-69815-8.

Publisher:
Sciencia Scripts
is a trademark of
Dodo Books Indian Ocean Ltd. and OmniScriptum S.R.L publishing group

120 High Road, East Finchley, London, N2 9ED, United Kingdom
Str. Armeneasca 28/1, office 1, Chisinau MD-2012, Republic of Moldova, Europe
Printed at: see last page
ISBN: 978-620-8-14298-8

I thank God first and foremost for the opportunity to realise yet another dream. Thank you to my loving family, my wife Adriana and my children Valentina and Vicente, who were often deprived of my presence due to the hours of study. Thank you to the preceptors, the teachers, the residents, Gabriel, Iaramim and Priscila, colleagues from the first Primary Health Care class. I would like to thank all the professionals at the UBS, my preceptor Janaíra and my supervisor André, who have been patient during this journey of exchange and learning.

SUMMARY

PRESENTATION

This book is the product of the Residency Conclusion Work of the lato-sensu postgraduate course with an emphasis on Primary Care of the Integrated Multiprofessional Health Residency at the Hospital de Clínicas in Porto Alegre, motivated by the resident's experience as a social worker in the Integrated Multiprofessional Health Residency Programme (RIMS), as well as previous experience as a Guardianship Councillor[1] . This experience influenced the investigation proposed in this research, which aims to bring to light the issue of violence against vulnerable groups, which is often invisible and/or "hidden" when not reported.

[1] TUTELAR COUNCIL: A permanent, autonomous, non-judicial body responsible for ensuring the fulfilment of children's and adolescents' rights, with attributions laid down in article 136 and article 98, where protective measures are applied whenever the rights of children and adolescents are threatened or violated (BRASIL, 1990).

CHAPTER 1

INTRODUCTION

Violence is currently considered one of the main problems experienced by the Brazilian population. Widely reported in the media and with high rates recorded by public services, violence has taken on a certain centrality in people's lives. Violence is the action of one human being against another caused by the abuse of force and power, or the omission of help when the other asks for it or needs it (MINAYO, 2014, p.39).

According to the Mortality Information System (SIM) of the Unified Health System (SUS), the threat to life is alarming, especially among young people, due to external causes such as accidents and violence, for example. Among adolescents aged 10 to 14, the causes of death due to aggression ranked second and in the 15 to 49 age group, first (BRASIL, 2013). Accidents accounted for 75.6% of all hospitalisations due to external causes, while violence accounted for 24.4%. Assaults accounted for the majority of hospitalisations due to violence (81.6%), followed by self-harm (19.4%) (BRASIL, 2010).

With specific reference to the advances made in social policies in the area of health over the last 30 years, the challenges of tackling violence as a public health issue are still many, especially when it comes to working to prevent, protect and promote health in the territory, which is the scene of power struggles, conflicts and contradictions, but also of potential, collective constructions with communities, health education and tackling violence.

Faced with the health impacts of violence, the Ministry of Health (MoH) has developed national information systems that make it possible, through compulsory notification forms for the various forms of violence, to identify the cases of which there is knowledge; to characterise and monitor the profile of violence according to the characteristics of the victim, the occurrence and the probable perpetrator of the violence; to identify risk and protection factors associated with the occurrence of violence; to identify areas most at risk of violence; and to identify the first referrals to the comprehensive care and protection network (BRASIL, 2011).

The purpose of the research proposed in this article is to bring to light the issue of violence against vulnerable groups, especially with regard to the process of compulsory notification of violence. However, it is well known that the lack of notification ends up making this problem invisible and/or hidden, despite the fact that in the case of children, adolescents, women and the elderly, the legislation makes it compulsory to fill in the compulsory notification form for violence. It was also identified that this issue is of total relevance in the work process of the multidisciplinary team in primary health care, debating the importance of compulsory notification of violence as an effective instrument for implementing public policies for victims of violence in the territory.

The main guiding principles of basic care, also known as primary care, are longitudinality: a personal relationship between the patient/user and professionals over time; first contact: the place users first seek care; comprehensiveness: guaranteeing health, all the health care the user needs and family orientation. The National Primary Care Policy prioritises family health as the strategy for expanding and consolidating primary care. One of the duties of primary care teams is to notify notifiable diseases and other illnesses and situations of local importance (BRASIL, 2012).

Notification of domestic violence, whether sexual or any other type of violence, was implemented in the Notifiable Diseases Information System (SINAN) by the Ministry of Health in 2009 and must be carried out compulsorily in situations of suspected or confirmed violence involving children, adolescents, women and the elderly, in compliance with Laws 8.069/90 (Statute of the Child and Adolescent), 10.741/03 (Statute of the Elderly) and 10.778/03 (Compulsory Notification of Violence Against Women).

The aim of this study was to identify the elements that influence the work of health professionals when it comes to compulsory reporting of violence. It aims to point out the possibilities and challenges for tackling violence in primary health care. The challenges for compulsory notification of violence to be understood from its legal consequences to the possibility of health promotion will be outlined below, given that the phenomenon of violence is part of the health/disease process.

The dialectical-critical method was chosen to guide all the phases of the study, from which this production was derived. Based on historical materialism, the main objectives of this method are to understand the interrelationships between phenomena and to search for their essence (TRIVINOS, 2007, p. 125).

The data was collected through semi-structured interviews with ten health professionals who make up the Family Health Strategy at the Santa Cecília UBS, linked to the HCPA. The research participants were health professionals who make up the Family Health Strategy (ESF), including two family doctors, a nurse, two nursing technicians, two community health workers, a nutritionist, a social worker and a pharmacist. The interviews were recorded with the interviewee's authorisation and carried out at the Basic Health Unit (UBS), in a suitable location that provided confidentiality and privacy. The information was analysed using technical content analysis according to Bardin. Content analysis is a set of methodological tools that are constantly being improved and applied to extremely diverse discourses (contents and continents) (BARDIN, 2011, p.15).

The recommendations of Resolution 466/12 were followed and approved by the Research Ethics Committee of the Hospital de Clínicas de Porto Alegre. All the interviewees were given a clear explanation of the study's objectives and signed the Free and Informed Consent Form (FICF) in two copies. The interviewees were also informed that they would be identified by letters and numbers in the order of the interviews (PS1, PS2, PS3...).

The theoretical framework for this research is systematised below. Two major aspects have been selected that enable the conceptual delimitation of the research's theoretical principles. Through this review, it is possible to broaden our knowledge of the phenomenon under study in order to subsidise future analyses. The typification of forms of violence and the role of primary care, together with health policy and the SUS, in tackling violence stand out.

CHAPTER 2

The typification of violence in Brazil and the ways of dealing with it

Brazil is one of the signatories of the United Nations Declaration of Human Rights, the World Health Organisation (WHO) and the Pan American Health Organisation on the issue of violence. In the WHO's World Report on Violence (2005), violence is defined as the intentional use of physical force or power, real or threatened, against oneself, against another person, or against a group in the community, that results in, or has a high likelihood of resulting in, injury, death, psychological harm, developmental disability or deprivation (WHO, 2005). According to Minayo (2006), violence in itself is neither a public health issue nor a traditional medical problem. However, it does have a decisive influence on people's health, as it can cause:

[...] death, physical injuries and traumas and countless mental, emotional and spiritual problems; it reduces the quality of life of people and communities; it requires a readjustment of the traditional organisation of health services; it poses new problems for preventive or curative medical care; and it highlights the need for much more specific, interdisciplinary, multi-professional, intersectoral and engaged action by the sector, aimed at the needs of citizens (MINAYO, 2006, p.45).

According to Minayo (2006), violence has affected public health in many ways, impacting on people's quality of life due to physical and psychological injuries, which is why integrated action from different areas of knowledge is needed in the public health sector, from the perspective of comprehensiveness[2] and intersectorality[3] , in order to respond to people's demands.

According to the definition given by the World Health Organisation (WHO), intrafamily violence is any action and/or omission that harms the well-being, physical or psychological integrity or freedom and the right to full development of a family member. Brazilian legislation protects children and adolescents, women and the elderly through specific legislation.

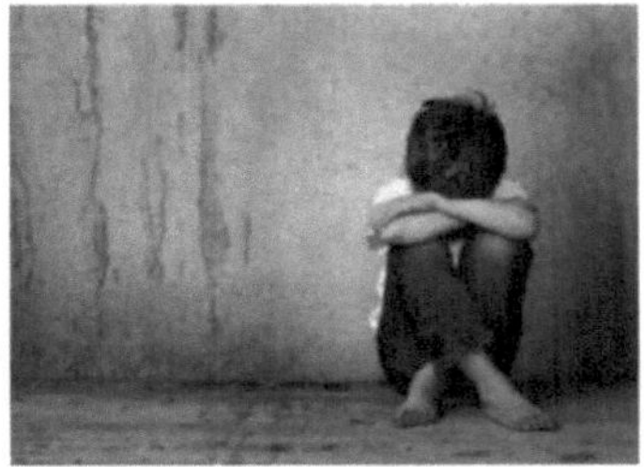

2.1 Violence against Children and Adolescents

With regard to children and adolescents, who are the weakest members of the family due to their peculiar condition as developing people, this segment has historically been the victim of crimes, basically due to society's omission. Even today, despite the existence of protective legislation, violations of rights against children and adolescents continue to occur, especially by those who should be caring for and protecting them, i.e. parents or guardians. According to the author:

The history of childhood is a nightmare from which we have recently

[2] Comprehensiveness, according to Article 198(II), gives the state the duty to provide comprehensive care, with priority given to preventive activities, without prejudice to assistance services in relation to the access that each and every citizen is entitled to.
[3] Intersectoral actions and the formation of networks to care for victims of violence are essential for carrying out actions to prevent and promote health and quality of life. (Brasil. Ministério da Saúde (MS), Plano Nacional de Enfrentamento da Violência Sexual contra crianças e adolescentes. Brasília: MS;2013).

begun to awaken. The further back we go in history, the lower the level of care for children, the greater the likelihood that they were murdered, beaten, terrorised and sexually abused (Guerra, 2001; p.53). As the author points out, we can see how cruel society has been to children. We only have to look at the history of children in Brazil since its discovery (1500) and colonisation (1530), when the first Portuguese expeditions arrived. Children and adolescents boarded the ships, heading for the new land, as orphans of the King, sent to Brazil to marry subjects of the Crown or even as passengers in the company of their parents, where they suffered all kinds of sexual abuse from the men on board. The orphans travelled under lock and key in order not to be raped, as they had to arrive in Brazil in a state of virginity in order to be accepted into marriage (ALBERTON, 2005). In Brazil, at the beginning of the 1980s, with the political opening at the end of the military dictatorship, some sectors of society began to question the way childhood was treated, proposing interventions that would bring children and adolescents closer to a set of rights. With the 1988 Constitution, children and adolescents came to be seen as subjects of rights and should be protected: It is the duty of the family, society and the state to ensure children and adolescents, with absolute priority, the right to life, health, food, education, leisure, vocational training, culture, dignity, respect, freedom, family and community life, as well as protecting them from all forms of neglect, discrimination, exploitation, violence, cruelty and oppression (BRASIL, 1988).

Article 227 of the constitution reformulates how children should be treated by the family, society and the state, considering them as subjects of law and no longer in an irregular situation. Protection becomes the responsibility of the family, society and the state, with absolute priority (ALBERTON, 2005). However, despite these advances, according to Volpi, it can be seen that children and adolescents in Brazil represent the group most exposed to rights violations by their families, the state and society, going against the perspective adopted by the 1988 Federal Constitution and complementary laws. Examples of this are: ill-treatment; sexual abuse and exploitation; exploitation of child labour; irregular adoptions, international trafficking and disappearances; hunger; extermination, torture and arbitrary arrests, which unfortunately still make up the scene where our children and adolescents parade. (VOLPI; 2008, p. 8)

In 1989, the United Nations Convention on the Rights of the Child (UN, 1989), in its article 19, declared that children should be protected against all forms of physical or mental violence, abuse or negligent treatment, maltreatment or exploitation, including sexual abuse, while they are in the custody of their parents, legal representative or any other person responsible for them. Brazil, as a signatory to this Convention, reaffirms in Article 227 of the Federal Constitution and in the Statute of the Child and Adolescent, the commitment to care, protection and the obligation for everyone to report cases of violence:

Art. 13 - Cases of suspected or confirmed ill-treatment of children or adolescents must be reported to the local Guardianship Council, without prejudice to other measures.

Art. 70 - It is everyone's duty to prevent the occurrence of threats or violations of the rights of children and adolescents.

Art. 245 - Failure by a doctor, teacher or person in charge of a health care establishment, primary school, pre-school or crèche to report to the competent authority any cases of which they become aware, involving suspicion or confirmation of ill-treatment of a child or adolescent. (Administrative Offence) (BRASIL, 1990).

As set out in the legislation, it is understood that the responsibility of the team and the health professional is to compulsorily notify the competent bodies, not just when there is evidence or confirmation, but also when there is a threat or suspicion, broadening the dimension of care beyond the consequences left by the violence, i.e. their care is also ensuring the protection of the victim and the prevention of violence. However, although many health professionals recognise this responsibility, the number of non-notifications is still very high. According to some studies, non-notification can be related to various factors such as overload of activities, deviation from duties, precarious conditions and difficulties in accessing basic equipment for exercising the profession, which leads to neglect of the information provided, including to the media (RICCA; OLIVEIRA, 2012, p.64). Although we recognise the efforts to understand violence as a public health issue, some authors point out that police stations are the first place to go to report violence, because the victims or those who deal with them do not consider the health sector to be competent to deal with this type of problem (NUNES; SALES, 2014, p.876). In this way, the failure of health professionals to report violence makes it invisible, especially when it comes to intrafamily violence, a phenomenon with cultural, social, economic and psychological factors.

In 2014, Law 13.010/14 was created, known as the Palmada Law, also known as the Menino Bernardo Law[4] . This law stipulates that the Federal Government, states and municipalities must work together to draw up public policies and implement actions aimed at curbing the use of physical punishment or cruel or degrading treatment and spreading non-violent forms of child education. Also according to the law, cases of suspected or confirmed physical punishment, cruel or degrading treatment or ill-treatment of children or adolescents must be reported to the nearest Guardianship Council. Finally, the reporting of abuse against children and adolescents is a phenomenon with major social repercussions and tackling it requires intersectoral action.

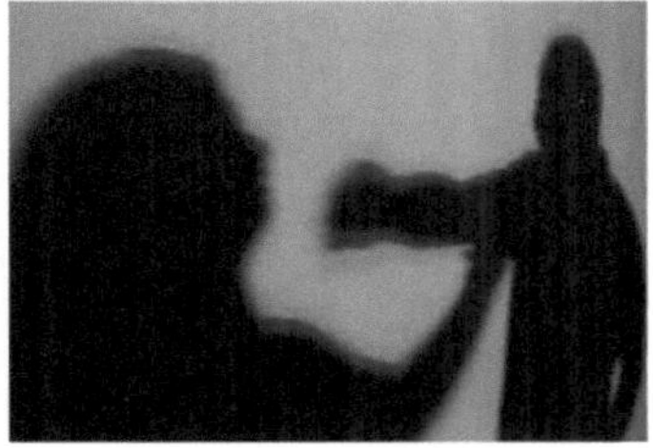

2.2Violence against Women

Like children and adolescents, women are also victims of violence because they are women in a society where macho culture predominates. Women have been heavily burdened and held responsible by this society, which imposes and determines their behaviour and role. According to Silva and Dal Prá: as far as family protection is concerned, this ends up overburdening women, as it is they who generally take on the role of carer for the two ends of the age pyramid, i.e. children and the elderly. (SILVA; DAL PRÁ, 2014, p.106). According to these authors, we can see how

[4] Law in honour of Bernardo Boldrini, the 11-year-old boy who was found dead in the city of Três Passos - RS, where the main suspects were his father and stepmother.

overburdened women are when they fulfil the role of carer on their own, and even when they work outside, having a double shift at home and in the market, and often being paid less. Institutional or state violence is also notorious when women are charged or made responsible as sole carers, who also need care and attention from social policies. Domestic violence is one of the types of violence against women that takes place in the home, in the family, with people who live in close proximity, but not necessarily family members, while intrafamily violence occurs between family members, but is not restricted to the physical space of the home (SAFFIOTI, 2001). Maria da Penha Law No. 11.340/2006 was created in honour of Maria da Penha Maia Fernandes, a victim of domestic violence in 1983, when she suffered two murder attempts by her ex-husband, the father of her three daughters. The first time she was shot in the back while she was asleep and the second when she tried to

electrocuting her in the bath, as a result of the aggressions she lost the movement in her legs and became a paraplegic. This law defines five forms of domestic violence against women:

Physical violence, understood as any conduct that offends bodily integrity or health;

Psychological violence, understood as any conduct that causes emotional harm and diminished self-esteem;

Sexual violence, understood as any conduct that forces you to witness, maintain or participate in an unwanted sexual relationship, through intimidation, threats, coercion or the use of force; that induces you to commercialise or use your sexuality in any way, that prevents you from using any contraceptive method or that forces you into marriage, pregnancy, abortion or prostitution;

Moral violence, understood as any conduct that constitutes slander, defamation or insult;

Property violence means any conduct that involves the retention, subtraction, partial or total destruction of objects, work tools, personal documents, goods, values and rights or economic resources, including those intended to meet their needs (BRASIL, 2006).

It's important to point out that the cases that go as far as murdering women are only the tip of the iceberg of violence against women, because as we saw earlier, women have suffered various types of violence simply because they are women, have historically been treated as objects, and have been disrespected and blamed. This gender violence has had a negative impact on society, creating myths and prejudices in social relations.

Femicide[5] is a heinous crime of cruelty that persists in our society. The city of Porto Alegre leads the way among the cities in the state of Rio Grande do Sul with the highest number of femicides, as illustrated in the graph below.

[5] Femicide or **feminicide** is a gender-based hate crime term widely defined as the murder of women, but definitions vary depending on the cultural context. (https://pt.wikipedia.org/wiki/Feminicídio)

Os crimes por cidade

Cidade	Crimes
Porto Alegre	48
Caxias do Sul	26
Alvorada	16
Viamão	16
Canoas	14
Novo Hamburgo	12
Pelotas	12
São Leopoldo	12
Santa Cruz do Sul	11
Santa Maria	10

TOTAL: 546
FEMINICÍDOS NO RS

177 em 10 municípios – Representa 32% do total

369 em 487 municípios – Representa 68% do total

Fonte: dados da Secretaria da Segurança Pública de 2012 a 2017

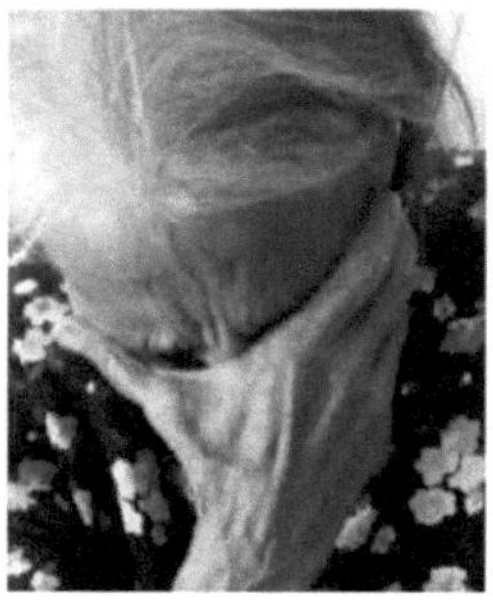

2.3 Violence against the Elderly

Intrafamily violence has spanned generations and the elderly population is also included in the statistics of victims of violence, especially when they cannot count on their primary network - the family and its social configurations (KERN, 2012); or they are victims of abandonment, neglect, mistreatment, property violence or other types of violence.

	CGVS/PMPA	DIAL 100
NEGLIGENCE	56,91%	68%
PHYSICS	35,96%	34%
PSYCHOLOGICAL	34,78%	59%
FINANCE	16,99%	40%
SUICIDE	13,00%	
SEXUAL	2,37%	1% (Minayo)

Source: CGVS/PMPA

According to the table above, neglect stands out as the main psychological violence against the elderly, according to Goldani:

[...] limited resources and childlessness are perhaps the most important reasons to explain why older people [...] can be neglected, forgotten or even abandoned. In societies where ownership rights exist, the absence of property can also lead to neglect (GOLDANI, 2004, p.229).

Goldani (2004) also warns of the risk of violence that elderly people can be exposed to when family care alternatives are exhausted. Situations like these have become increasingly common in many households, not only in families in situations of social vulnerability, but also in families with privileged socio-economic conditions, but without family support for their elderly members.

Issues related to family support and mistreatment of the elderly require qualified attention from health and social teams, as well as a collective effort to deal with them, including the availability of public resources to protect the elderly and assist them fully (BERNARDO; ASSIS, 2014). On 27 July 2011, a decree was passed amending Law 10.741 of 1 October 2003, the Statute of the Elderly, which determines the compulsory notification of acts of violence committed against the elderly in public or private establishments. The text defines **acts of violence against the elderly as "any action or omission committed in a** public or private place that causes death, harm or physical or psychological suffering.

Making health services responsible for classifying violence against the elderly facilitates the reporting of these aggressions, which helps to plan and implement public policies for this segment of the population, which is growing rapidly in our country. IBGE estimates for the next 30 years indicate that the elderly population will exceed 50 million people, reaching around 28 per cent of the population (Revista dos Direitos da Pessoa Idosa/SDH. Brasília/DF, 2011.)

According to the IBGE, there has been an increase in the number of elderly people, a vulnerable population that is therefore exposed to situations of violence, especially intra-family violence, such as children, adolescents and women. Therefore, the responsibility of health services in terms of typifying violence is also fundamental in primary care, in terms of tackling the various types of violence.

CHAPTER 3

The role of primary health care in tackling violence

When approaching intrafamily violence, as well as violence against children and adolescents, women and the elderly in terms of primary health care, it can be seen that this area plays an important role in recognising these types of violence. This is because it allows the team to get closer to the issues surrounding violence, it acts as the gateway to the system and is a reference point for the user's first contact.

The main guiding principles of basic care, also known as primary care, are longitudinality: a personal relationship between the patient/user and professionals over time; first contact: the place where users first seek care; comprehensiveness: guaranteeing health, all the health care the user needs and family orientation.

The National Primary Care Policy prioritises family health as a strategy for expanding and consolidating primary care. One of the duties of primary care teams is to notify diseases and illnesses of compulsory notification and other illnesses and situations of local importance (BRASIL, 2012).

Among the competences of primary health care, it is worth highlighting territorial actions of articulation, partnerships and health promotion with families and the community. These actions are guided by policies, including the National Primary Care Policy (PNAB), created in 2012 with the aim of legitimising the implementation of the Organic Health Law in primary care throughout the country;

[...] by a set of health actions, both individual and collective, which include health promotion and protection, disease prevention, diagnosis, treatment, rehabilitation, harm reduction and health maintenance, with the aim of developing comprehensive care that impacts on the health situation and autonomy of people and on the determinants and conditioning factors of the health of communities. (BRASIL, 2012, p. 19). When mentioning disease prevention, the National Primary Care Policy (PNAB) relates social determinants of health as a health/disease process that seeks to articulate the different dimensions of life, considering historical, economic, social, cultural, biological and other aspects. In this sense, the National Humanisation Policy of the SUS proposes the Expanded Clinic (BRASIL 2004), which moves away from the notion of health as the absence of symptoms and broadens the concept of care to include the related social determinants of health and illness. In this way, health also means happiness, self-esteem, security, satisfactory relationships and stability in the world of work (BENEDETTO; SILVEIRA, 2013, p.73). The authors present the expanded concept of health with feelings that are opposed to violence, i.e. the victim of violence is a sad, depressed, insecure, fearful and threatened person, in aggressive relationships, and there is also a relationship between violence and the economic crisis and social inequality in which the country lives.

Recognising the social and economic impact of violence on the SUS, the Ministry of Health implemented the National Policy for Reducing Morbidity and Mortality from Accidents and Violence in 2001.

In 2006, through the Secretariat of Health Surveillance (SVS), it implemented the Violence and Accident Surveillance Programme (VIVA) within the SUS. The following year, Brazilian municipalities became part of this programme, with the adoption of the notification form for domestic, sexual and other violence. Alongside this form, an Instructable[6] was created, which aims to help health professionals, when assisting people who are victims of violence, to fill in the form in a standardised way, providing guidance and helping to qualify the notification (MINISTÉRIO DA SAÚDE, 2011).

However, this tool for tackling violence, which makes it possible to map places where violence occurs, its victims and aggressors, as well as the implementation of public policies, has encountered difficulties in its realisation.

Faced with these difficulties, it is necessary for the multidisciplinary team to be attentive to issues of care for victims of violence, without omitting cases to be reported. In this sense, the actions of the professional, together with the team, can contribute to tackling situations of violence when they broaden their concept of care, not naturalising situations of violence or making it invisible in primary health care when it is not reported.

[6] This manual is a data collection tool published by the Ministry of Health for filling in the Notification/Individual Investigation Form for Domestic, Sexual and/or Other Violence. Its aim is to help health professionals and professionals from other sectors who work in services that assist people who have suffered or are living in situations of violence to fill in the form in a more standardised way.

CHAPTER 4

RESULTS AND DISCUSSION

Analysing the data collected from the health professionals interviewed, we identified various aspects of the reality of the phenomenon under study, which are presented below in three main themes:

"Materialised violence: finding out how to report it";

"Knowledge about compulsory notification of violence in Primary Health Care";

"Compulsory notification of violence: the responsibility of a single professional or a team?".

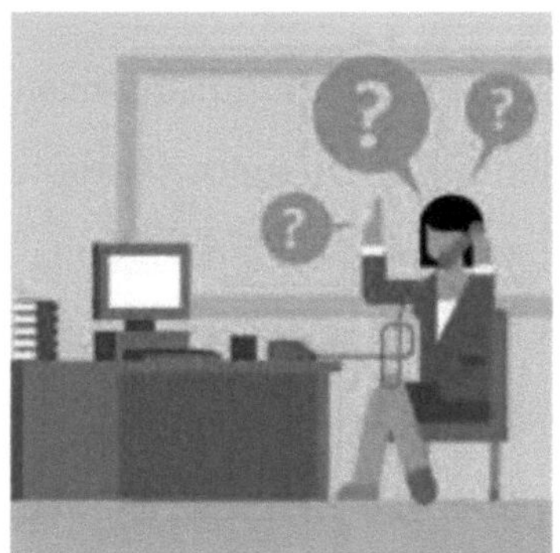

4.1 Violence materialised: Check to report

It was possible to identify that health professionals are unclear about the concept of violence, which directly implies their behaviour in relation to notification when violence is suspected and/or found. As such, both working with cases of violence and reporting them become challenges for PHC work, as it is essential for professionals to recognise their demands, including situations of violence, and to be able to propose intervention strategies.

> *"Whether or not I get to see it, I share with the other colleagues in the team." (PS 1)*

> *"But I think we end up working more on this concreteness. When it's physical violence, the* other types of violence still get *overlooked." (PS 5)*
>
> *"We need to work harder on our technical approach to assessing what is in fact violence and what is not. I think intentionality is one of the guiding principles for me to conceptualise violence" (PS 10).*

According to Chaui, the myth of non-violence in Brazilian society acts as a foundation for the mythical construction of a good society, one, undivided, peaceful and orderly. This raises the image of a generous, joyful, sensual, supportive people who are unaware of racism, sexism and homophobia, who respect ethnic, religious and political differences, who live without prejudice because they don't discriminate against people because of their ethnicity, social class or sexual, religious or professional choices. But how can the myth of Brazilian non-violence persist under the impact of real, everyday violence, known to all, and currently amplified by its dissemination and diffusion by the mass media (CHAUI, 2017)?

The author answers this question about the myth of non-violence through a set of ideological mechanisms that affirm and deny the presence of violence in our society, including the inversion of reality, which allows violent behaviours, ideas and values to be concealed as if they were non-violent. The author gives an example: male chauvinism is seen as protection for the natural fragility of women, which includes the idea that women need to be protected from themselves, because, as everyone knows, rape is a feminine act of provocation and seduction; white paternalism is seen as protection to help the natural inferiority of blacks and indigenous people; repression against homosexuals is seen as natural protection for the sacred values of the family and, now, for the health and life of the entire human race threatened by AIDS brought by the degenerate (CHAUI, 2017, p.37).

Health professionals therefore need to recognise violence as a current, multifaceted and extremely challenging phenomenon. In order to deal with any type of violence, it is first necessary to recognise its existence. Recognising intra-family violence, for example, can help to minimise the damage caused to each family (SHIMBO AY et al, 2011).

According to the interviews, the majority of professionals believe that compulsory notification of violence should only be made after prior assessment and exhaustion of the team's enquiries into the situation:

> *"As I work with a group of professionals: psychologists, nutritionists, doctors, nurses, technicians... at first, when we feel this demand for a group, we talk about it, and from there, we try to decipher if it's really happening". (PS 1)*
>
> *"It would be better to investigate the situation and go to the patient's home too, because sometimes they don't speak, they have difficulties. Trying to reach them in some way. Firstly to get them to trust you. So that takes a while..." (PS 3)*
>
> we always *try to assess; to assess personally, by making a visit, by attending, by talking to the person, talking to the family, and assessing what is really behind that suspicion or that report from the team or the school, if there really is a situation of violence, if there is an aggressor." (PS 10).*

Professionals don't feel safe in situations of violence. The expressions *"decipher" and "ascertain"* are words that are antagonistic to suspicion -

although there is doubt, there is still a need for certainty, for this violence to materialise. For health professionals, *"decipher"* has the meaning of unravelling, discovering, revealing; and *"investigate"* has *the* meaning of ascertaining, making sure. It's as if the professionals denied it at first and only understood confirmed *and/or* verified situations as violence in order to notify them.

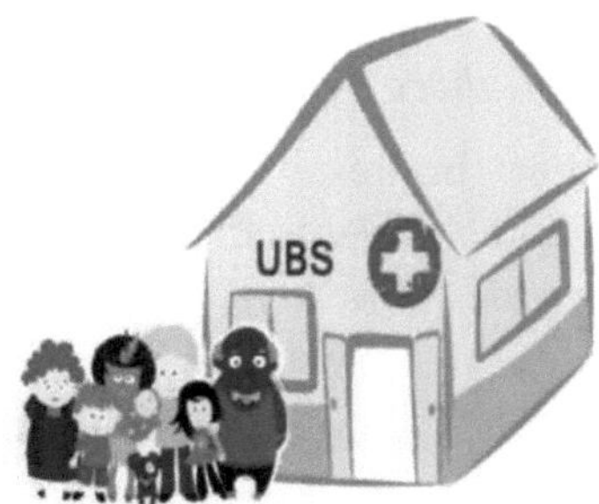

4.2 Knowledge about compulsory notification of violence in PHC.

With regard to knowledge of compulsory notification, although they have a certain amount of experience, the professionals showed limited knowledge of how to fill in the notification form and to which bodies cases of violence should be reported. The fragmented way in which work is managed and organised means that the division of tasks by professional category favours the lack of notification.

Notification is for epidemiological purposes and follows an internal process within Public Health, serving to build profiles through the Notifiable Diseases Information System - SINAN, which will be used to build more effective public policies. External communication should be sent to the bodies in the protection network (Women's Police Station, Public Prosecutor's Office or Judiciary, Guardianship Council, Municipal Council for the Elderly, among others).

Based on the reports below, it is clear that the majority of professionals understood compulsory notification as a complaint, while few identified it as an epidemiological record of violence in the territory through the SINAN form. The professionals' understanding of the flow of compulsory notification at the UBS was also unclear.

> *"There's the SINAN notification form, which we notify in writing, and we notify by calling the relevant bodies, there's the Guardianship Council, there's the*
>
> CRAM, there are these other bodies that provide assistance and report violence, and by discussing this in a *multi-professional team, everyone can help in these cases." (PS 4)*
>
> *"Yeah, I know it exists, but I don't know where to look for it, I don't know how it's filled in, who it's sent to after it's been filled in. I don't know, I think the team could do with some training on this". (PS 6)*
>
> *"(...) we have a flow for those who work at the UBS, (...) but it's not very clear, because I went to ask my colleagues and no one could tell me." (PS 7) "I took a course last year on compulsory notification, I know there's a form, that every time we notice any kind of violence, it's not just physical, it's verbal." (PS 8) (PS 8)*
>
> *"We have SINAN in primary care, but I confess it's little used, I hardly ever use it, I end up forgetting about SINAN". (PS 10)*

It was also noted that compulsory notification was never mentioned as mandatory in situations of violence against children, women and the elderly, or as an advance in legislation in Brazil to protect historically victimised populations and, therefore, its importance. Notification is a doubly important instrument in the fight against violence, as it brings benefits to individual cases and is an instrument for the epidemiological control of violence (GONÇALVES; FERREIRA, 2002).

According to Monteiro (2010), the procedure that has generally been carried out in health units is characterised by the receipt of a complaint, identification or suspicion, the filling in of a compulsory notification form and, in some cases, the preparation of a report to the competent bodies in order to refer the case. However, it is still difficult for health professionals in primary health care to formalise the compulsory notification of violence. Studies have shown that it is difficult for health professionals to identify and notify cases, and that these practices are still incipient at the level of the care network, occurring casually and unsystematically (LUNA;

FERREIRA; VIEIRA, 2010; MOREIRA et al., 2013). These findings highlight the mismatch between what is proposed by legal provisions and public policies to tackle the problem and the actual practice of health professionals, especially in primary health care.

In terms of knowledge, the health professionals say they recognise the gap in training and suggest training and continuing education on the subject:

> *"During university I remember seeing it* briefly, but where I went deeper was in the *multi-professional residency* training*" (PS 4);*
>
> *"There was no thought given to my training" (PS 5);*
>
> *"It would be up to mditc edu to provide ongoing education to the team" PPS 6);*
>
> *"I think in the multiprofessional seminars we could perhaps work on rich cases" (PS 9),*

There is also limited knowledge about compulsory notification of violence in primary care. Some professionals became familiar with the notification routine after taking a training course:

> *"I think that this compulsory notification should be publicised to all employees, because I'm sure that many colleagues don't even know where the form is, or where it is, that there is a folder, which I didn't even know existed until I took this course" (PS 8).*

Continuing education can be understood as work-based learning, i.e. it takes place in the daily lives of people and organisations. It is based on the problems faced in reality and takes into account the knowledge and experience that people already have. It proposes that health workers' education processes should be based on problematising the work process, and considers that workers' training and development needs should be guided by the health needs of people and populations. The aim of continuing health education processes is to transform professional practices and the organisation of work itself (BRASIL, 2009).

In addition to the suggestion of ongoing education on the subject, the professionals also raise concerns about the link when it comes to reporting:

> *caente has to be very careful before saying something like that" (PS 1).*
>
> *"The priority is to welcome this family, to listen, to give this support" (PS 2).*
>
> *"Prímaim consegmirque clon trust you. It takes a while, but that's how it goes" (PS 3).*
>
> *"Look, this family needs to be seen too, they need to be heard, what's going on" (PS 5).*

In the speeches, the importance of this bond between professional and patient is evident. Closeness and the ability to be welcoming, binding, responsible and resolute are fundamental to making primary care effective as the preferred contact and gateway to the Unified Health System (SUS). The bond consists of building relationships of affection and trust between users and health professionals (BRASIL 2012).

Concern about breaking the bond with the patient/user is one of the reasons why health professionals in primary care don't report incidents, which is often related to complaints. The health professional is afraid of losing the bond with the patient and compromising care and treatment at the health unit. However, the professional/patient bond requires a dialogue of complicity and co-responsibility, and the professional needs to take ownership of this instrument in order to fulfil their ethical duty to notify and inform the patient of the importance of this record as a subsidy to the manager in implementing public policies in the territory.

What stands out in the professionals' speeches is their concern for the family, which needs to be listened to and welcomed. The act of notifying is not simply about judging, blaming or holding the family responsible; on the contrary, the family needs support, especially from the state, so that it can fulfil its role as carer and protector, but unfortunately, there is still denial and loss of rights, especially in the current situation, where familism can be considered a trigger for violence when family care becomes basically feminist, confined to private life (MIOTO , 2015, p.89).

Therefore, we cannot expect the family alone to cope with complex situations such as violence, a phenomenon inherent to human beings, but the legislation is clear about everyone's responsibility and the need to strengthen a support network for families to deal with the issue of violence, drawing attention to the importance of intersectoral support (JUNIOR et al., 2017).

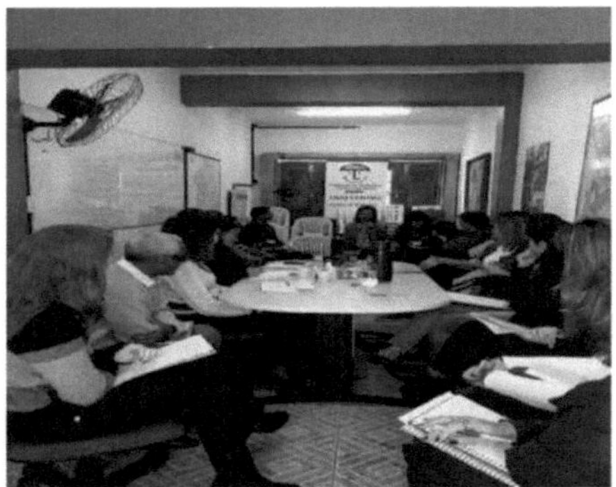
Intersectoral network meeting

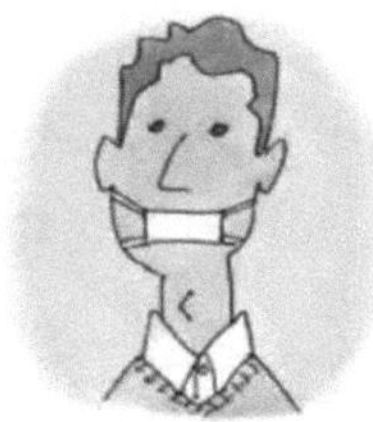

4.3 Compulsory Notification of Violence: The responsibility of a single professional or the team?

Violence, as a multifactorial phenomenon, requires multi-professional and interdisciplinary approaches, and no single professional category is expected to deal with such complex situations. According to Vasconcelos (2012), it would be difficult for just one professional to deal with all aspects of such a complex reality, which is why comprehensive care requires multi-professional work.

Specifically, intra-family violence, as the subject of compulsory notification, calls on everyone: the state, civil society, health education institutions and healthcare organisations to act on two levels. The first is prevention by guaranteeing access. The second, psychosocial care for families in situations of violence, so that they can maximise their material and symbolic resources and thus reinvent their relationships, breaking the cycle of intrafamily violence (MOREIRA; SOUZA, 2012).

It was noted from the health professionals' statements that situations of suspected and confirmed violence are demands on the team, although some health professionals recognise their legal responsibility and seek to provide the team with tools. This attitude apparently "frees" the person who identified the violence from responsibility and involvement, so it is essential that health professionals assume a position of responsibility for the cases identified, through teamwork and liaison between the other services that deal with situations of violence (SILVA PA et al, 2009).

It was found that the decision to notify is not guided by legislation, but by aspects of professional experience, structure and articulation of the protection network. This behaviour, expressed in the professionals' statements, is confirmed in the literature in relation to the factors that can influence non-notification in primary health care: such as proximity to the territory, fear of confidentiality on the part of the professionals. (ROLIM, et al. 2014, p.802)

> *"Imagine a nurse at the reception desk filling in the SINAN form and putting her stamp and name on it. She's going to make home visits in the area and what guarantee does she have that her name will remain confidential? So these issues of safety for the professional are very much linked to non-notification in primary care (...) it's complicated, because it's very easy for the aggressor or the population to identify who made the notification, because the primary care worker is in that person's home and territory every day" (PS 10).*

According to the above statement, despite the fact that it is compulsory for health professionals to report, there is no guarantee of confidentiality or protection of the integrity of the whistleblower. This ends up causing professionals to be reluctant to make such a report for fear of reprisals or threats (MONTEIRO, 2010). In this way, it is possible to infer that the phenomenon of violence ends up taking precedence over protection, in other words, the permeability of insecurity, as an expression of violence, is gaining more space in the social fabric.

According to Garbin (2014), it is essential that health professionals have broad and consistent knowledge of the problem of violence in order to fulfil their ethical and legal role. They must therefore officially report suspected or confirmed cases of violence against children, adolescents and older adults to the relevant bodies,

with a view to preventing the problem, monitoring and protecting victims.

In this sense, the notification of suspicions and/or findings should be considered as prevention in the context of primary care, as strategies to guarantee the rights of the population. The information produced by notification also favours the visibility of the phenomenon, which is essential for planning actions to prevent and deal with violence, as it makes public policies more effective.

With regard to the work of the multidisciplinary team in primary care, when it comes to situations of violence, the importance of this approach is evident in the statements made by health professionals:

> *"At a team meeting we discussed what had happened and the team agreed that this should be sent to a network group, our network, where the girl would have better care with psychologists, social workers, in short a whole group (PS 2).*
>
> *"As a professional, I've never (worked) alone, I've always*

been accompanied and sought out other colleagues so that I could work together, given how complex it is" (PS 5).

"(...) there are different types of violence, with different types of approaches. When the demand comes from the team, when the team makes a referral, the situation is not always a situation of violence, or a situation of neglect or mistreatment" (PS 10).

According to the health professionals, situations of violence are shared, demanded and discussed in multidisciplinary team meetings and from an intersectoral perspective, meeting the objectives of primary care as a coordinator of care (PNAB, BRASIL, 2012). Intersectoral actions and the formation of networks for the care of victims of violence are essential for carrying out actions to prevent and promote health and quality of life (GARBIN CAS *et al.* 2014, p.1885).

It can also be seen that multi-professional teamwork is a potential way of dealing with situations of violence in primary care, a favourable space for discussing violent cases and events, as well as formalising care flows. Dealing with violence is extremely complex, which is why it requires a multidisciplinary approach, the existence of a protocol, systematic dialogue between professionals about the problem, formal meetings, group discussions, factors that can contribute to the notification process and to overcoming the characteristics of isolated, disjointed acts that are the sole responsibility of each professional (SILVA PA et al. 2009, p.61).

However, multi-professional care is not enough; there needs to be integration and articulation between the different professions, in other words, interdisciplinary work to deal with complex situations involving intrafamily violence. Eichherr and Cruz emphasise the importance of multi-professional work in tackling violence and the articulation of the intersectoral network, as well as the involvement of professionals from this network in acting in cases of violence as a strategy for coping, changing social reality and, essentially, as a form of care (EICHHER and CRUZ, 2017).

Networking has been one of the main strategies for tackling violence in primary health care. Situations and cases of violence are discussed at intersectoral meetings in the region, with referrals and follow-up to services that assist families in situations of violence. Thus, health professionals understand the importance of this networking based on their work as a multi-professional and interdisciplinary team, i.e. different areas engaging in dialogue with their knowledge with common objectives.

However, health professionals who are part of a multi-professional team need to be trained in how to report violence. According to the information collected, they suggest ongoing education in team meetings about violence, understanding that it should be recognised, integrated into the health area and everyone's responsibility, as it affects people's living conditions and quality of life. In this sense, notification becomes a strategy for tackling intrafamily violence when responsibility for protecting children and adolescents, women and the elderly is shared with other sectors of society.

CHAPTER 5

FINAL CONSIDERATIONS

This study showed that compulsory notification of violence in primary care still encounters obstacles. For health professionals, one of the main challenges to compulsory notification is their limited knowledge about notification and communication. The training of professionals, who in their reports recognise the existing gap and suggest training and continuing education on the subject. The multidisciplinary approach and working from an intersectoral perspective are seen as potential in tackling violence in primary health care.

Compulsory notification is not a police report. Its purpose is to subsidise actions to prevent and deal with violence, as well as the implementation of public policies for victims. And this needs to be a constant among the team. The misinformation and lack of knowledge among health professionals has to do with the understanding of the phenomenon of violence, which is often seen as a cause outside the health area, i.e. exclusively a case of public security. Compulsory notification, as a strategy for dealing with violence, enables intersectoral work, which is essential in primary health care as a coordinator of care.

Despite the team's limitations, there are potentials and possibilities for tackling violence in primary care, as it is a privileged space for welcoming, identifying, attending to, reporting and monitoring situations of violence, based on the Family Health Strategies (ESF), for example.

This form of teamwork makes it possible to hold meetings to discuss cases, provide matrix support and provide training for professionals, including in situations of violence, in which there is success in evaluations with the multidisciplinary approach and work from an intersectoral perspective, but also that the duty of health professionals is to develop strategies aimed at overcoming the obstacles to compulsory notification of violence and contribute to greater visibility of the problem in primary health care.

In the case of the phenomenon of violence, through compulsory notification, a coordinated intervention between sectors and social policies is decisive for fully meeting the health needs of the population that uses the SUS. In this way, health promotion, protection and rehabilitation start to look at other aspects of the reality that make up the health/disease process.

CHAPTER 6

BIBLIOGRAPHY

ALBERTON, Mariza Silveira. **Child rape: abominable crimes: humiliate, hurt, torture and kill!** Porto Alegre: AGE, 2005.

BARDIN, L. **Content Analysis. Lisbon,** Portugal; Edições 70, LDA, 2009.

BENEDETTO, Elisa Scherer; SILVEIRA, Esalba. **Soil and roots of the individual, social and programme dimensions of vulnerability and the seeds in the child health process.** Textos e Contextos (Porto Alegre), v.12, n.1,p.68 - 84, jan./jun.2013

BARDIN, **Lawrence. Content analysis.** São Paulo: Edições 70, 2011.

BRAZIL. **1988 Constitution of the Federative Republic of** Brazil. Brasília, DF: Senate, 1988.

BRAZIL. Federal Law No. 8.0690/90. **Statute of the Child and Adolescent (ECA).** Federal Official Gazette 1990; 16 and 27 July.

BRAZIL. Law No. 10.741, of 1st October 2003. Provides for the **Statute of the Elderly** and other Provisions. Federal Official Gazette 2003; 3 Oct.

BRAZIL. Law No. 10.010/14. **Palm Law,** of 27 June 2014.

BRAZIL. Federal Law No. 11340/06. **Maria da Penha Law.** Federal Official Gazette 2006; 7 Aug.

BRAZIL. Federal Law No. 8.080/90 - **Unified Health System (SUS).** Official Gazette

Official Gazette 1990; 19 Sep.

BRAZIL. **Ministry of Health. National Health Council. Resolution no. 466,** of 12 December 2012.

BRAZIL. **Ministry of Health. Health Care Secretariat. Department of Primary Care. National Primary Care Policy/ Ministry of Health. Health Care Secretariat. Primary Care Department.** - Brasília: Ministry of Health, 2012. 110p.:il. -

(Series E. Health Legislation)

BRAZIL. Ministry of Health. **National Policy for Permanent Education in Health.** Brasília, 2009, p. 20

BRAZIL - **Ministry of Health. Instructions for completing the Individual Notification/Investigation of Domestic, Sexual and/or Other Violence in the Notifiable Diseases Information System - SINAN NET.** - Brasília: Ministry of Health, 2011.

BRAZIL. **Secretariat for Human Rights of the Presidency of the Republic: Manual for confronting violence against the elderly. It is possible to prevent. It is necessary to overcome it.** / Secretariat for Human Rights of the Presidency of the Republic; Text by Maria Cecília de Souza Minayo. - Brasília, DF: Secretariat for Human Rights of the Presidency of the Republic, 2014. 90p.

CHAUI, Marilena. **On Violence** / Marilena Chaui; organisers Ericka Marie Itokazu, Luciana Chaui-Berlink. -1. Ed. Belo Horizonte: Autêntica Editora, 2017.

EICHHERR, L.M; CRUZ, L.R. **Violence against children and adolescents: (in)visibilities and problematisations**. SI UNISC, Santa Cruz do Sul, Vol. 1, n. 1, Jul./Dec. 2017, p.<85-87>.

GARBIN, C.A.S; DIAS I.A; ROVIDA, T.A.S; GARBIN, A.J.I. **Challenges for health professionals in the notification of violence: compulsory, effective and referral**. Ciência & Saúde Coletiva,. p.1879-1890, 2014.

GOLDANI, A.M. **Intergenerational relations and the reconstruction of the welfare state: why should this relationship be rethought for Brazil?** In: CAMARANO, A.A (eds.). The new Brazilian elderly far beyond 60? Rio de Janeiro: IPEA, 2004.

GUERRA, Viviane Nogueira de Azevedo. **Parental violence against children: the tragedy revisited.** 4. ed. rev. and expanded. São Paulo: Cortez 2001.

IBGE. **Brazilian Institute of Geography and Statistics (IBGE 2010)**

JUNIOR, G.B.S; ROLIM, A.C.A; MOREIRA, G.A.R; CORREA, C.R.S; VIEIRA, L.J.E. **Trabalho e Educação em Saúde. Rio de Janeiro**, v 15 n. 2,

2017, p. 469-484.

KERN, F.A. **Mediations in networks as a methodological strategy for social work.** Porto Alegre: Edipucrs, 2012.

LUNA, G. L. M.; FERREIRA, R.C.; VIEIRA, L.J.E.S. **Notification of child and adolescent abuse by Family Health Team professionals.** Ciência & Saúde Coletiva, Rio de Janeiro, v. 15, n. 2, p. 481-491, 2010

MINAYO, Maria Cecília de Souza. **Violence and Health.** Rio de Janeiro: Editora Fiocruz, 2006. 132 p. (Themes in Health Collection).

MINAYO, Maria Cecília de Souza. **The challenge of knowledge: qualitative research in health.** São Paulo: Hucitec, 2007.

MIOTO, R. C.; CAMPOS, M. S.; CARLOTO, C. M. (Orgs.). **Familism, rights and citizenship: contradictions in social policy.** São Paulo: Cortez, 2015. 248 p.

MOREIRA, M.I.C; SOUZA, S.M.G. **Intrafamily violence against children and adolescents: private space to the public scene. O Social em Questão** - Year XV - n° 28, 2012.

MOREIRA, G. A. R. et al. **Instrumentation and knowledge of family health team professionals on the notification of child and adolescent abuse.** Revista Paulista de Pediatria, São Paulo, v. 31, n. 2, p. 223-230, 2013.

NUNES, A.J; SALES M.C.V. **Violence against children in the Brazilian scenario.** Free Themes. 2014, p.871- 880.

Health policy today: interfaces & challenges in the work of social workers / organisation Marco José de Oliveira Duarte...[et al.].--1.ed.-- Campinas, SP: Papel Social, 2014. **Article 15: Elderly health and comprehensive care** (Maria Helena de Jesus Bernardo; Mônica de Assis).

Journal of the Rights of the Elderly/SDH. Brasília/DF, 2011

RICCA, Anna Elisa T. de Oliveira; OLIVEIRA, Bernadete de. **Unveiling Paths: The underreporting of accidents and violence against the elderly.** Revista Portal de Divulgação. 2012, p.64-76

SAFFIOTI, Heleieth I.B. **Feminist contributions to the study of gender violence.** In Cadernos Pagu, n.16, 2011, p.11-136.

SILVA, Adriana; DAL PRÁ, Keli Regina. **Population ageing in Brazil: the place of families in protecting the elderly.** Argumentum, Vitória(ES), v.6,n.1,p.99-115,jan./jun.2014.

SILVA, P.A; LUNARDI, V.L; SILVA, M.R.S; LUNARDI Filho W.D. **A Notificação da Violência Intrafamiliar Contra Crianças e Adolescentes na percepção dos Profissionais de Saúde**, Cienc Cuid Saude; 2009,p.56-62.

SHIMBO, A.Y; LABRONICI L.M; MANTOVANI M.F. **Reconhecimento da violência intrafamiliar contra idosos pela equipe da Estratégia Saúde da Família**, Esc Anna Nery (impr.)2011, p.506-510.

TRIVINOS, A.N.S. **Introdução à Pesquisa em Ciências Sociais: a pesquisa qualitativa em educação.** São Paulo: Atlas, 2007.

VASCONCELOS, A. M. A **prática do serviço social: cotidiano, formação e alternativas na área da saúde.** 8. ed. São Paulo: Cortez, 2012.

VOLPI, M. **O adolescente e o ato infracional/** Mário Volpi(org.).-7.ed.- São Paulo: Cortez, 2008.

http://www2.portoalegre.rs.gov.br/portal_pmpa_novo/

https://pt.wikipedia.org/wiki/Feminicidio

CHAPTER 7

ANNEX- SINAN form

República Federativa do Brasil
Ministério da Saúde

SINAN
SISTEMA DE INFORMAÇÃO DE AGRAVOS DE NOTIFICAÇÃO
FICHA DE NOTIFICAÇÃO INDIVIDUAL

Nº

Caso suspeito ou confirmado de violência doméstica/intrafamiliar, sexual, autoprovocada, tráfico de pessoas, trabalho escravo, trabalho infantil, tortura, intervenção legal e violências homofóbicas contra mulheres e homens em todas as idades. No caso de violência extrafamiliar/comunitária, somente serão objetos de notificação as violências contra crianças, adolescentes, mulheres, pessoas idosas, pessoa com deficiência, indígenas e população LGBT.

Dados Gerais

1 Tipo de Notificação — 2 - Individual

2 Agravo/doença — VIOLÊNCIA INTERPESSOAL/AUTOPROVOCADA — Código (CID10) Y09

3 Data da notificação

4 UF

5 Município de notificação — Código (IBGE)

6 Unidade Notificadora — 1- Unidade de Saúde 2- Unidade de Assistência Social 3- Estabelecimento de Ensino 4- Conselho Tutelar 5- Unidade de Saúde Indígena 6- Centro Especializado de Atendimento à Mulher 7- Outros

7 Nome da Unidade Notificadora — Código Unidade

8 Unidade de Saúde — Código (CNES)

9 Data da ocorrência da violência

Notificação Individual

10 Nome do paciente

11 Data de nascimento

12 (ou) Idade — 1 - Hora 2 - Dia 3 - Mês 4 - Ano

13 Sexo — M - Masculino F - Feminino I - Ignorado

14 Gestante — 1-1ºTrimestre 2-2ºTrimestre 3-3ºTrimestre 4- Idade gestacional ignorada 5-Não 6- Não se aplica 9-Ignorado

15 Raça/Cor — 1-Branca 2-Preta 3-Amarela 4-Parda 5-Indígena 9- Ignorado

16 Escolaridade — 0-Analfabeto 1-1ª a 4ª série incompleta do EF (antigo primário ou 1º grau) 2-4ª série completa do EF (antigo primário ou 1º grau) 3-5ª à 8ª série incompleta do EF (antigo ginásio ou 1º grau) 4-Ensino fundamental completo (antigo ginásio ou 1º grau) 5-Ensino médio incompleto (antigo colegial ou 2º grau) 6-Ensino médio completo (antigo colegial ou 2º grau) 7-Educação superior incompleta 8-Educação superior completa 9-Ignorado 10- Não se aplica

17 Número do Cartão SUS

18 Nome da mãe

Dados de Residência

19 UF

20 Município de Residência — Código (IBGE)

21 Distrito

22 Bairro

23 Logradouro (rua, avenida,...) — Código

24 Número

25 Complemento (apto., casa, ...)

26 Geo campo 1

27 Geo campo 2

28 Ponto de Referência

29 CEP

30 (DDD) Telefone

31 Zona — 1 - Urbana 2 - Rural 3 - Periurbana 9 - Ignorado

32 País (se residente fora do Brasil)

Dados Complementares

Dados da Pessoa Atendida

33 Nome Social

34 Ocupação

35 Situação conjugal / Estado civil — 1 - Solteiro 2 - Casado/união consensual 3 - Viúvo 4 - Separado 8 - Não se aplica 9 - Ignorado

36 Orientação Sexual — 1-Heterossexual 2-Homossexual (gay/lésbica) 3-Bissexual 8-Não se aplica 9-Ignorado

37 Identidade de gênero: — 1-Travesti 2-Mulher Transexual 3-Homem Transexual 8-Não se aplica 9-Ignorado

38 Possui algum tipo de deficiência/ transtorno? — 1- Sim 2- Não 9- Ignorado

39 Se sim, qual tipo de deficiência /transtorno? — 1- Sim 2- Não 8-Não se aplica 9- Ignorado

- Deficiência Física
- Deficiência Intelectual
- Deficiência visual
- Deficiência auditiva
- Transtorno mental
- Transtorno de comportamento
- Outras ______

Dados da Ocorrência

40 UF

41 Município de ocorrência — Código (IBGE)

42 Distrito

43 Bairro

44 Logradouro (rua, avenida,...) — Código

45 Número

46 Complemento (apto., casa, ...)

47 Geo campo 3

48 Geo campo 4

49 Ponto de Referência

50 Zona — 1 - Urbana 2 - Rural 3 - Periurbana 9 - Ignorado

51 Hora da ocorrência (00:00 - 23:59 horas)

52 Local de ocorrência — 01 - Residência 02 - Habitação coletiva 03 - Escola 04 - Local de prática esportiva 05 - Bar ou similar 06 - Via pública 07 - Comércio/serviços 08 - Indústrias/construção 09 - Outro ______ 99 - Ignorado

53 Ocorreu outras vezes? — 1 - Sim 2 - Não 9 - Ignorado

54 A lesão foi autoprovocada? — 1 - Sim 2 - Não 9 - Ignorado

SVS 15.06.2015

Violência

55 Essa violência foi motivada por: 01-Sexismo 02-Homofobia/Lesbofobia/Bifobia/Transfobia 03-Racismo 04-Intolerância religiosa 05-Xenofobia 06-Conflito geracional 07-Situação de rua 08-Deficiência 09-Outros ______ 88-Não se aplica 99-Ignorado

56 Tipo de violência 1- Sim 2- Não 9- Ignorado
- Física
- Psicológica/Moral
- Tortura
- Sexual
- Tráfico de seres humanos
- Financeira/Econômica
- Negligência/Abandono
- Trabalho infantil
- Intervenção legal
- Outros ______

57 Meio de agressão 1- Sim 2- Não 9- Ignorado
- Força corporal/ espancamento
- Enforcamento
- Obj. contundente
- Obj. pérfuro-cortante
- Substância/ Obj. quente
- Envenenamento, Intoxicação
- Arma de fogo
- Ameaça
- Outro ______

Violência Sexual

58 Se ocorreu violência sexual, qual o tipo? 1- Sim 2 - Não 8 - Não se aplica 9- Ignorado
- Assédio sexual
- Estupro
- Pornografia infantil
- Exploração sexual
- Outros ______

59 Procedimento realizado 1- Sim 2 - Não 8 - Não se aplica 9- Ignorado
- Profilaxia DST
- Profilaxia HIV
- Profilaxia Hepatite B
- Coleta de sangue
- Coleta de sêmen
- Coleta de secreção vaginal
- Contracepção de emergência
- Aborto previsto em lei

Dados do provável autor da violência

60 Número de envolvidos
1 - Um
2 - Dois ou mais
9 - Ignorado

61 Vínculo/grau de parentesco com a pessoa atendida 1-Sim 2-Não 9-Ignorado
- Pai
- Mãe
- Padrasto
- Madrasta
- Cônjuge
- Ex-Cônjuge
- Namorado(a)
- Ex-Namorado(a)
- Filho(a)
- Irmão(ã)
- Amigos/conhecidos
- Desconhecido(a)
- Cuidador(a)
- Patrão/chefe
- Pessoa com relação institucional
- Policial/agente da lei
- Própria pessoa
- Outros ______

62 Sexo do provável autor da violência
1 - Masculino
2 - Feminino
3 - Ambos os sexos
9 - Ignorado

63 Suspeita de uso de álcool
1- Sim
2 - Não
9- Ignorado

64 Ciclo de vida do provável autor da violência:
1-Criança (0 a 9 anos)
2-Adolescente (10 a 19 anos)
3-Jovem (20 a 24 anos)
4-Pessoa adulta (25 a 59 anos)
5-Pessoa idosa (60 anos ou mais)
9-Ignorado

Encaminhamento

65 Encaminhamento: 1-Sim 2-Não 9-Ignorado
- Rede da Saúde (Unidade Básica de Saúde,hospital,outras)
- Rede da Assistência Social (CRAS, CREAS, outras)
- Rede da Educação (Creche, escola, outras)
- Rede de Atendimento à Mulher (Centro Especializado de Atendimento à Mulher, Casa da Mulher Brasileira, outras)
- Conselho Tutelar
- Conselho do Idoso
- Delegacia de Atendimento ao Idoso
- Centro de Referência dos Direitos Humanos
- Ministério Público
- Delegacia Especializada de Proteção à Criança e Adolescente
- Delegacia de Atendimento à Mulher
- Outras delegacias
- Justiça da Infância e da Juventude
- Defensoria Pública

Dados finais

66 Violência Relacionada ao Trabalho
1- Sim 2 - Não 9 - Ignorado

67 Se sim, foi emitida a Comunicação de Acidente do Trabalho (CAT)
1- Sim 2 - Não 8 - Não se aplica 9- Ignorado

68 Circunstância da lesão
CID 10 - Cap XX

69 Data de encerramento

Informações complementares e observações

Nome do acompanhante | Vínculo/grau de parentesco | (DDD) Telefone

Observações Adicionais:

TELEFONES ÚTEIS

Disque Saúde - Ouvidoria Geral do SUS	Central de Atendimento à Mulher	Disque Direitos Humanos
136	180	100

Notificador

Município/Unidade de Saúde | Cód. da Unid. de Saúde/CNES

Nome | Função | Assinatura

Violência interpessoal/autoprovocada Sinan SVS 15.06.2015

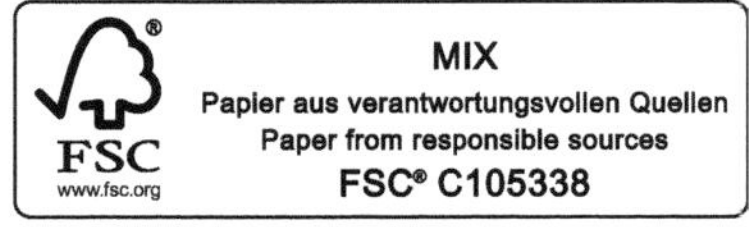

Printed by Books on Demand GmbH, Norderstedt / Germany